Author

Born on a crisp autumn day in 1966, Chihauna's life has been a testament to the strength of the human spirit. Raised by a single mother, Chihauna developed a profound appreciation for family values from a young age. Her mother, a hardworking and compassionate individual, instilled in her a sense of responsibility and a deep love for those around her.

At the heart of Chihauna's world are her four children, two grandbabies, and her devoted husband of over two decades. Family gatherings at the Hunter household are filled with love, laughter, shared stories, and the warmth that can only come from years of unconditional love. Chihauna's dedication to her family is unwavering, and she cherishes every moment spent with her loved ones.

In 2018, Chihauna faced a life-altering challenge when she experienced a stroke. Where she had to learn to walk and talk again. Determined to overcome the odds, she embarked on a journey of recovery that showcased her resilience and indomitable spirit. The stroke not only strengthened her but also redirected her focus towards a healthier lifestyle.

As part of her recovery and newfound commitment to well-being, Chihauna discovered the transformative power of natural juicing. This revelation became a passion that she now shares with others. Chihauna's kitchen is a vibrant hub of fruits and vegetables, where she crafts delicious and nutritious juices, each sip a celebration of vitality and healing.

Chihauna's compassion extends beyond her family. She has become a source of inspiration for others facing health challenges, offering guidance and support to those on similar paths. Her advocacy for the benefits of natural juicing has become a beacon of hope for many.

A two-time published author, Chihauna has channeled her experiences into words, penning books that resonate with authenticity and wisdom. Her writings not only delve into her personal journey but also serve as guides for those navigating their own trials.

In addition to her literary pursuits, Chihauna has a creative side that finds expression in Semi-Precious Gemstones beaded jewelry. Her intricate designs reflect her zest for life and the vibrant colors that surround her. Each piece tells a story, mirroring the diverse chapters of Chihauna's rich and multifaceted life.

Chihauna's love for life extends to her love for travel. From the serene landscapes of coastal retreats to the bustling markets of exotic cities, Chihauna finds joy in exploring the world with her husband. These adventures not only provide cherished memories but also serve as a reminder of the boundless possibilities' life has to offer.

As Chihauna celebrates her 57th year, she stands as a beacon of love, resilience, and the transformative power of embracing life's challenges. Her journey, marked by family, health, creativity, and compassion, leaves an indelible mark on those fortunate enough to know her. Chihauna's story is a testament to the extraordinary heights one can reach with an unwavering faith, spirit, and a heart full of love.

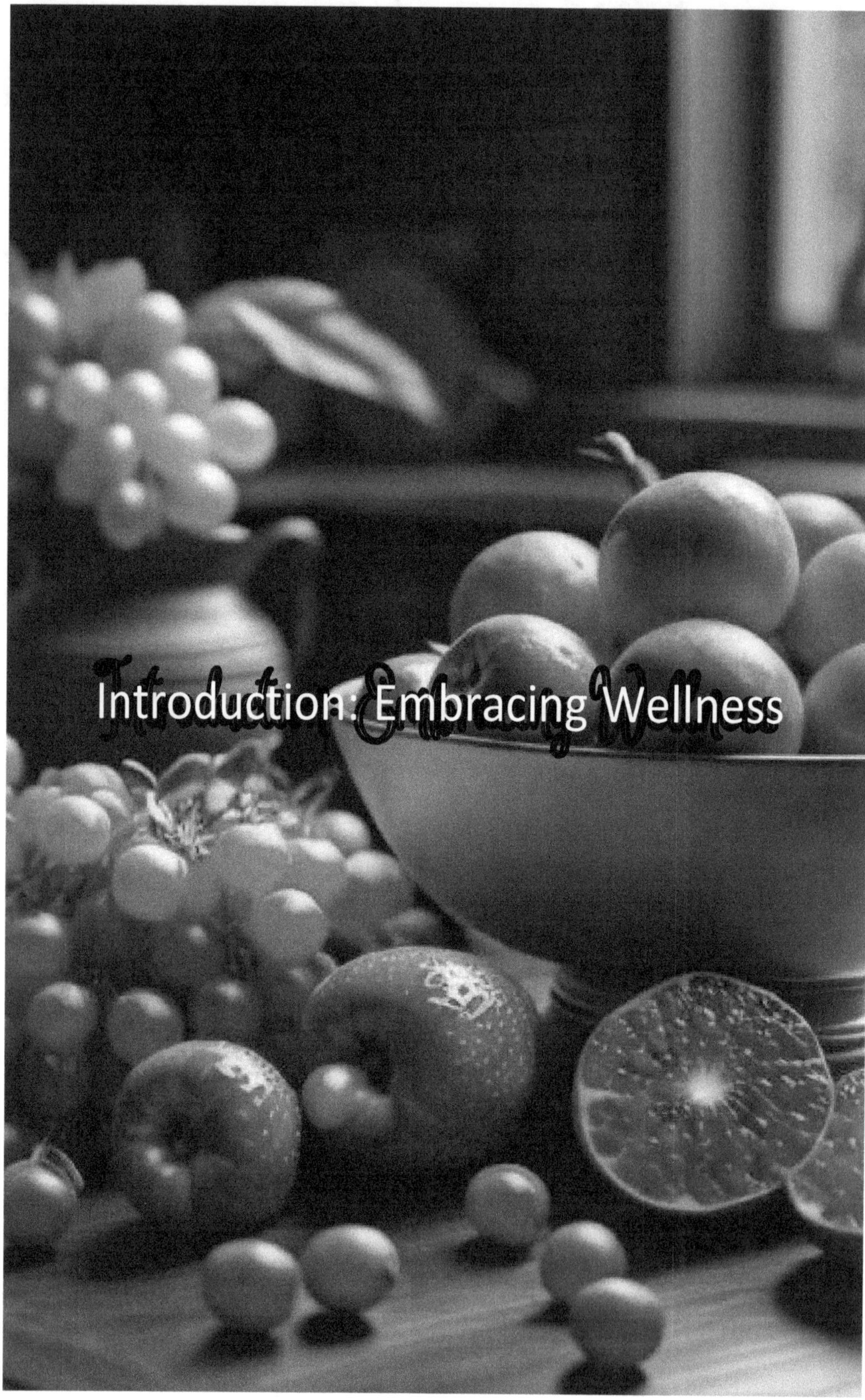

Introduction: Embracing Wellness

Welcome to a journey of self-discovery, growth, and wellbeing. It's easy to overlook the importance of our health and happiness. This Journey is a heartfelt exploration of the various facets of wellness, aimed at guiding you toward a more balanced, fulfilling life.

In the pages that follow, we will delve into the realms of physical health, mental clarity, emotional resilience, and spiritual harmony. We'll explore practical strategies, insightful reflections, and inspiring stories to help you cultivate a sense of purpose, inner peace, and vibrant energy.

Our goal is not to provide a one-size-fits-all solution but rather to empower you with knowledge and tools to craft your path to wellness. Whether you are seeking ways to improve your fitness, enhance your mental focus, or nurture your relationships, this journey is to meet you where you are and guide you toward where you want to be.

Remember, wellness is not a destination but a continual, evolving process. It's about embracing the journey, celebrating small victories, and learning from setbacks. By the end of this exploration, we hope that you will find inspiration, motivation, and practical steps to lead a life that is not only healthy and vibrant but also deeply fulfilling.

So, without further ado, let's embark on this transformative odyssey together. Here's to your health, happiness, and the discovery of your best self.

Table of Content

Table of Content

Week 4:
Day 22: Cultivating Positive Habits
Day 23: Practicing Mindfulness
Day 24: Cultivating Compassion
Day 25: Embracing Hope
Day 26: Cultivating Mindful Habits
Day 27: Practicing Self Reflection
Day 28: Cultivating Gratitude
Day 29: Setting Intentions for Growth
Day 30: Celebrating Your Achievements

This journey should provide a comprehensive guide to cold press juicing over the next 30 days.

Conclusion

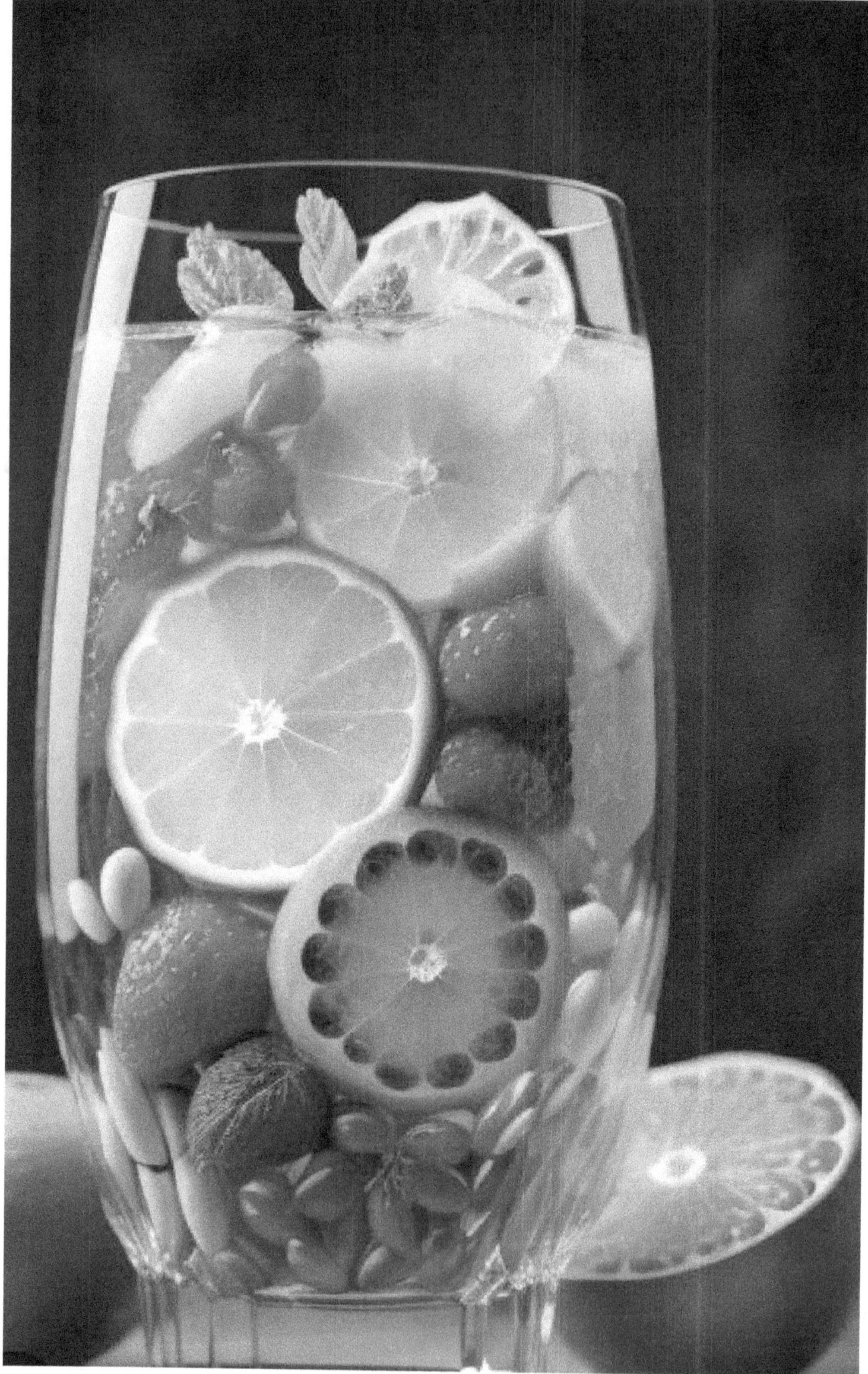

Day 1: Benefits of Cold Press Juicing
Welcome to Day 1 of your 30-day cold press juicing journey!
Today, let's dive into the incredible benefits of cold press juicing:

1. **Nutrient Retention:** Cold press juicers operate at low speeds, minimizing heat and oxidation. This process helps retain essential vitamins, minerals, and enzymes present in fruits and vegetables, providing you with the most nutritious juice possible.

2. **Better Taste and Quality:** Cold press juices have vibrant flavors. The slow juicing process preserves the natural taste of ingredients, creating a refreshing and enjoyable drinking experience.

3. **Improved Digestibility:** Cold press juices are easier to digest compared to whole fruits and vegetables. When you remove the fiber during juicing, your body can absorb nutrients more efficiently, promoting better digestion and nutrient absorption.

4. **Boosted Immunity:** Cold press juices can be packed with immune-boosting vitamins like vitamin C. Drinking regularly can strengthen the immune system, helping your body fight off sickness, bacteria, and infections.

5. **Detoxification:** Cold press juicing helps your body with the detoxification processes. The abundance of antioxidants in fresh

juices helps to eliminate toxins and promote a healthier, clearer complexion.

6. **Maximized Energy Levels:** The high concentration of vitamins and minerals in cold press juices provides a natural energy boost. Say bye-bye to midday slumps and hello to sustained energy throughout the day.

7. **Weight Management:** Cold press juice, that is made with vegetables, can be low in calories and very beneficial as far as your nutrients are concerned. When you introduce juicing into your diet, it can help you with your weight management.

As you embark on this 30-day journey, keep these benefits in mind. Cold press juicing is not just a trend; it's a lifestyle choice that can transform your health and well-being. Get ready to experience a refreshing and revitalizing way to nourish your body! Stay tuned for more exciting juicing insights and recipes throughout the month.

Day 2: Cold Press Juicer Types and Features

Welcome to day 2! Today let us explore the different types of cold press juicers, and their features to help you make an informed choice:

1. **Masticating Juicers:**
   - Operation: Masticating juicers work by crushing and squeezing fruits and vegetables to extract juice. They operate at slow speeds, preserving nutrients and preventing oxidation.
   - Features: These juicers are versatile and can manage a wide range of produce, including leafy greens, nuts, and even wheatgrass. They are efficient at extracting the juice and producing a higher yield compared to other juicer types.
2. **Hydraulic Press Juicers:**
   - Operation: Hydraulic press juicers use thousands of pounds of pressure to extract juice from fruits and vegetables. They are often used in commercial settings for large-scale juice production.
   - Features: These juicers yield very dry pulp, indicating efficient juice extraction. They are excellent for juicing hard and soft produce, making them suitable for a variety of recipes.

Key Features to Consider:
   - **Speed:** Cold press juicers operate at slow speeds (typically, 80 RPM or lower), minimizing heat generation and oxidation for nutrient-rich juices.

- **Versatility:** Look for juicers with a wide feeding chute, allowing you to juice whole or large pieces of fruits and vegetables without extensive preparation.
- **Ease of Cleaning:** Consider juicers with dishwasher-safe parts and designs that are easy to disassemble and clean. This feature makes cleanup a breeze after your juicing sessions.
- **Durability**: Choose a juicer made from high-quality, durable materials to ensure long-lasting performance and reliability.

Understanding these juicer types and features will empower you to select the best juicer for your needs. Whether you are a fan of green juices, vibrant fruit blends, or nutrient-packed nut milk. Your chosen juicer will play a large role in your juicing experience. Stay tuned for more exciting juicing insights and recipes tomorrow!

Happy juicing! □□□

Day 3: Choosing the Right Ingredients for Your Juices

Welcome to day 3! Today let us explore the art of choosing the perfect ingredients for your cold press juices. Selecting the right fruits and vegetables not only ensures delicious flavors but also maximizes the health benefits of your juices.

Here is how to make the best choices:

1. **opt for Fresh and Organic:**
   - Choose fresh, ripe, and organic produce whenever possible. Choosing Organic can help you with cleaner, healthier juice.

2. **Embrace Variety:**
   - Include a wide selection of colorful fruits and vegetables in your juices. Each color represents different nutrients, so a diverse range ensures you are getting a wide array of vitamins and minerals.

3. **Balance Sweet and Savory:**
   - Balance the sweetness of fruits with the earthiness of vegetables. This combination not only enhances the flavor but also moderates the sugar content,
   making your juices more balanced and nutritious.

4. **Include Delicious Greens:**
   - kale, spinach, and Swiss chard are immensely powerful in nutrition They can be extraordinarily rich and beneficial in vitamins, minerals, and antioxidants. Add a handful of leafy greens to your juices for an instant nutrient boost.

5. **Experiment with Herbs:**
   - Fresh herbs like mint, basil, and parsley can add unique flavors to your juices. They also come with their own set of health benefits and can elevate the taste of your creations.

6. **Mindful Pairings:**

- Some ingredients complement each other exceptionally well. For example, apple pairs wonderfully with kale, and citrus fruits like oranges or lemons can enhance the flavors of various vegetables.

7. **Seasonal Juicing:**

- Experiment with seasonal produce. Not only is it fresher and more flavorful, but it also allows you to enjoy a variety of ingredients throughout the year. By being mindful of your ingredient choices, you can create juices that are not only tasty but also incredibly beneficial for your health. So, head to your local market, explore the seasonal offerings, and get creative with your cold press juicing! Stay tuned in for more juicing tips and recipes tomorrow.

Happy juicing! □□□

Day 4: Cold Press vs. Centrifugal Juicers: Pros and Cons

Welcome to day 4! Today let us unravel the differences between cold press and centrifugal juicers.

Understanding the pros and cons of each category will enable you to make a well-informed choice when deciding.

Pros:

- **Nutrient Preservation:** Cold press juicers operate at low speeds, minimizing heat generation. This slow process helps preserve delicate enzymes and nutrients, resulting in healthier juices.
- **Higher Yield:** Cold press juicers extract more juice from fruits and vegetables, ensuring you get the most out of your ingredients.

- Versatility: They can handle a wide variety of produce, including leafy greens, hard vegetables, and even nuts, making them versatile for various recipes.

Cons:

- **Price:** Cold press juicers are more expensive upfront. However, their efficiency and nutrient retention often justify the investment for health-conscious individuals.

Centrifugal Juicers:

Pros:

- **Speed:** Centrifugal juicers operate at high speeds, making them faster than cold press juicers. They are ideal for those who want quick, on-the-go juicing.
- **Affordability:** Centrifugal juicers are usually more budget-friendly, making them a popular choice for beginners or those on a tight budget.

Cons:

- **Nutrient Loss:** Due to the high speed and heat generated during the juicing process, centrifugal juicers may lead to some nutrient loss and oxidation.
- **Limited with Leafy Greens:** They might not be as effective at juicing leafy greens and softer fruits compared to cold press juicers.

Choosing the Right Juicer:

- **Consider Your Needs:** If you prioritize maximum nutrition and versatility, a cold press juicer is the way to go. If speed and budget are more crucial for you, a centrifugal juicer might be a suitable choice.
- **Long-Term Health Investment:** While cold press juicers might be more expensive at first, consider them as an

investment in your long-term health. The nutrient-rich juices they produce can contribute significantly to your overall well-being. Gaining insight into the distinctions among these juicer types assists you in selecting one that aligns with your lifestyle and health goals. Stay tuned for more juicing insights and tips tomorrow!

Happy juicing!

□□□

Day 5: How to Clean and Maintain Your Cold Press Juicer

Welcome to Day 5! Today, let us talk about a crucial aspect of juicing - cleaning and maintaining your cold press juicer. Keeping your juicer in top condition ensures it functions efficiently and produces high-quality juices every time. Here is a guide to help you clean and maintain your cold press juicer:

Cleaning Your Cold Press Juicer:

1. **Unplug the Juicer:** Always start by unplugging your juicer to ensure safety during the cleaning process.

2. **Disassemble the Juicer:** Take apart your juicer carefully, following the manufacturer's instructions.

Most cold press juicers are easy to disassemble.

3. **Rinse Immediately:** After juicing, rinse the parts under warm water immediately. This prevents pulp and residue from drying out, making the cleaning process much easier.

4. **Use a Cleaning Brush:** Most juicers come with specialized cleaning brushes. Use it to gently scrub the mesh screen, auger, and other components. The brush helps remove stubborn pulp and fiber.

5. **Avoid Soap on Mesh Screen:** While other parts can be washed with mild soap, avoid using soap on the mesh screen.
Instead soak the screen in warm water and gently brush off any remaining pulp.

6. **Inspect for Residue:** Double-check all components to ensure no residue remains. Pay extra attention to small crevices and corners where pulp can hide.

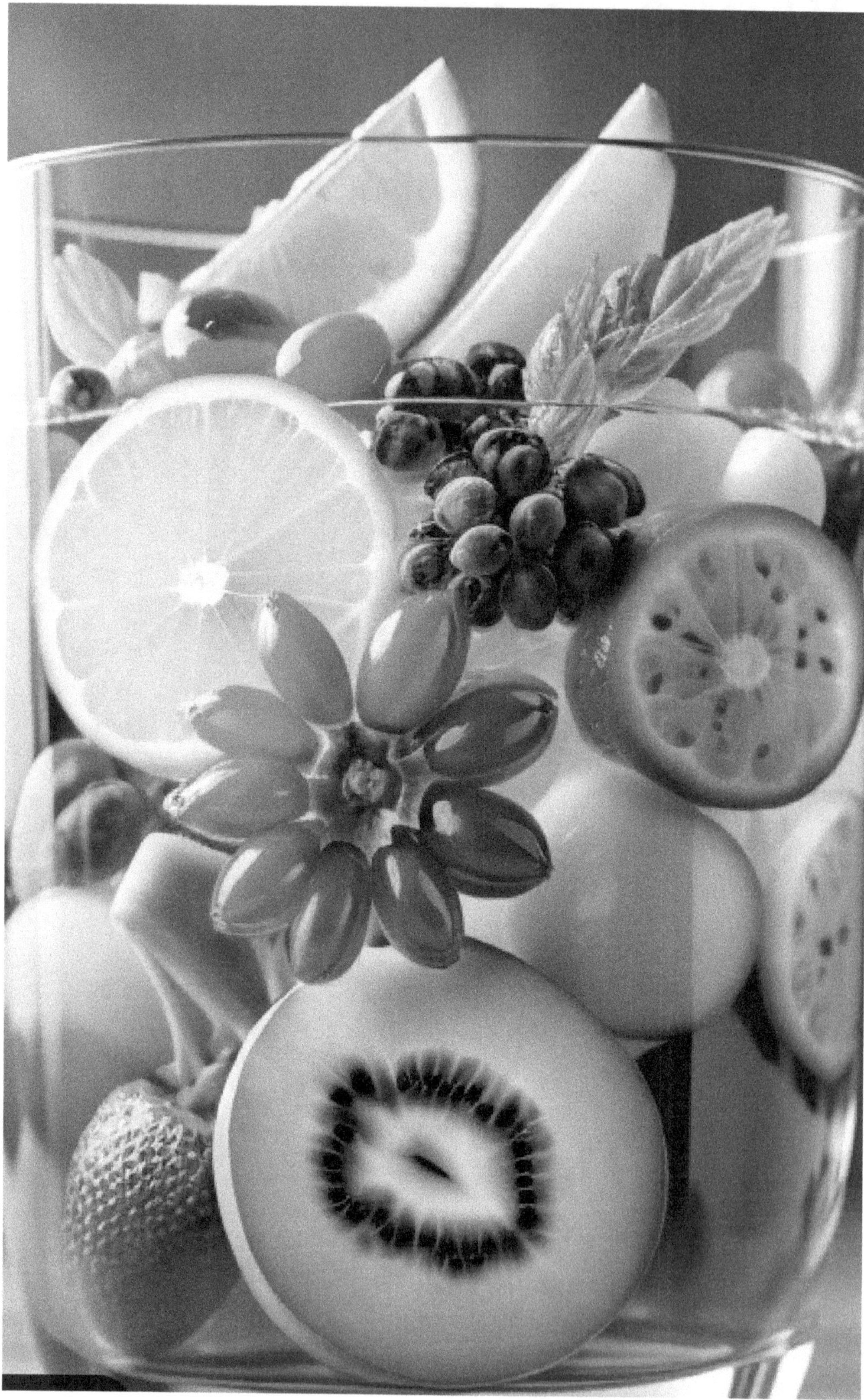

Maintaining Your Cold Press Juicer:

1. **Regular Oil Application:** Some juicers have parts that require occasional lubrication. Refer to your user manual to know which parts need food-grade lubricating oil and apply it as recommended.

2. **Avoid Overloading:** Be mindful not to overload a juicer with too many fruits or vegetables at once.

Overloading can strain the motor and affect the juicer's efficiency.

3. **Rotate Produce:** When juicing, rotate soft and hard produce to ease the juicing process. For example, follow a leafy green with harder vegetables like carrots to help push through the greens effectively.

4. **Clean Immediately After Use:** Prompt cleaning prevents pulp and juice residues from drying, making the cleaning process simpler and quicker.

By following these cleaning and maintenance practices, you will ensure your cold press juicer stays in excellent condition, providing you with fresh and nutritious juices every time you use it. Stay tuned for more juicing tips and exciting recipes tomorrow!

Happy juicing! □□□

Day 6: Beginner-Friendly Cold Press Juice Recipes

Welcome to day 6! Today let us kick-start your juicing experience with a few beginner-friendly and delicious cold press juice recipes. These recipes are easy to make and perfect for those new to juicing. Grab your fresh ingredients and let us get to juicing!

Green Fusion Bliss:

Ingredients

- 1 green apple
- green grapes
- 1 cucumber a handful of spinach
- 2 stalks of Celery
- a piece of ginger pineapple

Directions:

1. Wash all your ingredients thoroughly.
2. Cut them into sizes that fit your juicer's chute.
3. Juice the apple, cucumber, spinach, pineapple, celery, and ginger.
4. Stir well and pour into a glass. Enjoy your refreshing green juice!

Golden Citrus Delightful

Ingredients

- 4 carrots
- 2 oranges
- 2 golden beets
- 1-inch piece of turmeric piece of ginger

Directions:

1. Juice the carrots, golden beet, ginger, turmeric, and oranges.
2. Mix the juices thoroughly.
3. Pour into a glass and savor the vibrant flavors of this carrot-orange is delightful!

Berrylicious:

Ingredients

- 1 fresh red beetroot
- 1 cup mixed berries (blueberries, strawberries, raspberries)
- a piece of ginger
- 1-2 tablespoons honey or agave syrup (optional for sweetness)

Directions:

1. Wash the berries and remove stems if necessary.
2. Juice the strawberries, beets, blueberries, ginger, and raspberries together.
3. Taste the juice and add honey or agave syrup if desired.
4. Mix well, and your colorful berry juice is ready to enjoy!

Minty Melon:

Ingredients

- cucumber cut into pieces
- 1/2 cup of mint leaves
- a lime
- watermelon
- 1-2 tablespoons honey (optional)

Directions:

1. Clean your cucumber and cut it into pieces.
2. Juice the cucumber, mint leaves, lime, and watermelon together.
3. Taste the juice and add honey if you prefer a sweeter taste.
4. Stir well and pour over ice for a refreshing cucumber-mint cooler.

These beginner-friendly juice recipes are packed with vitamins and minerals, making them a delightful and nutritious way to begin your juicing journey.

Experiment with different ingredients and find the flavors that suit your taste buds best. Stay tuned for more juicing tips and inspiration tomorrow!

Happy juicing! □ □ □

Day 7: Tips for Storing Cold Press Juices

Welcome to day 7! As you continue your juicing journey, it is essential to know how to store your precious creations properly. Today, let us explore some valuable tips for storing your cold press juices to maintain their freshness and nutritional value.

1. **Use Airtight Containers:**
   - Transfer your freshly made juice into airtight glass containers or bottles. Avoid plastic containers, as they can leak chemicals into the juice.
2. **Fill to the Top:**
   - Fill the container to the top to minimize air exposure. The less air in the container, the slower the oxidation process, preserving the juice's nutrients.
3. **Add Citrus:**
   - If your juice contains citrus fruits like lemon or lime their natural acidity can help preserve the juice. Consider adding a splash of lemon or lime juice to your recipes for both flavor and longevity.
4. **Refrigerate Immediately:**
   - Place your juice in the refrigerator immediately after juicing. Cold temperatures slow down the degradation of nutrients and maintain freshness.
5. **Consume Quickly:**
   - Cold press juices are best consumed fresh. Try to drink your juices within 24 to 48 hours to enjoy maximum flavor and nutritional benefits.

6. **Freeze for Longevity:**
   - If you have made a large batch, you can freeze the leftover juice in ice cube trays. Put the frozen juice cubes into a freezer bag. When you are ready to drink, simply thaw a few cubes in the refrigerator and mix them with fresh juice.

7. **Shake Well Before Drinking:**
   - Cold press juices might naturally separate overtime. Give the container a good shake before drinking to ensure an even distribution of flavors and nutrients.

8. **Store Properly for Travel:**
   - If you need to take your juice on the go, use an insulated cooler bag with ice packs to keep the juice cold and fresh.

By following these storage tips, you can extend the shelf life of your cold press juices while preserving their health benefits. Now that you know how to store your juices effectively, you can enjoy the convenience of having nutritious, homemade juices readily available. Stay tuned for more juicing insights and exciting recipes tomorrow!

Happy juicing! □□□

Day 8: The Power of Green Juices

Welcome to day 8! Today let us delve into the incredible world of green juices and explore the numerous health benefits they offer. Green juice is packed with lots of nutrients that can transform your health and well-being.

Why Green Juices?

1. **Because they are full of rich Nutrients:** Green vegetables like as spinach, kale, and Swiss chard are packed with an abundance of vitamins A, C, and K, as well as minerals like iron and calcium. These nutrients are vital for maintaining overall health.

2. **Alkalizing Properties:** Many green vegetables have alkalizing effects on the body, helping balance its pH levels. A balanced pH is linked to better digestion, increased energy, and reduced risk of chronic diseases.

3. **Detoxification:** Chlorophyll, the pigment that gives greens their color, is a natural detoxifier. It helps cleanse the liver and eliminate toxins from the body, promoting a healthier system.

4. **Boosted Immunity:** Green vegetables can be a good source of antioxidants, which can strengthen your immune system and aid your body in fighting off bacteria, infections, and illnesses.

5. **Improved Digestion:** Green juice not only tastes good and good for you, but it is an excellent provider of dietary fiber supporting digestion and promoting a healthy gut. A healthy digestive system is essential for nutrient absorption and overall well-being.

Green Goddess

Ingredients

• handful of spinach

• 1 cucumber

• 1 green apple

• 1 lemon

• hand full of cilantro

• 1-inch piece of ginger

Directions:

1. Clean all your ingredients thoroughly.
2. Cut them into sizes that fit your juicer's chute.
3. Juice spinach, cucumber, green apple, lemon, cilantro, and ginger.
4. Stir well and pour into a glass. Feel the revitalizing power of this Green Goddess Elixir!

Embrace the power of green juices in your daily routine. Their vibrant flavors and health-boosting properties make them a wonderful addition to your juicing repertoire. Stay tuned for more juicing tips and exciting recipes tomorrow!

Happy juicing!

□□□

Day 9: Green Juice Recipes for Detoxification

Welcome to day 9! Today let us focus on green juice recipes specifically designed for detoxification. Detoxifying your body can help eliminate toxins, boost your energy, and promote overall well-being. Here are two refreshing and detoxifying green juice recipes to try:

Cleansing Green Citrus Juice:

Ingredients

- 2 cups kale leaves
- 1 cucumber
- 2 green apples
- 1 lemon
- 1-inch piece of ginger
- fresh mint leaves

Directions:

1. Wash all the ingredients thoroughly.
2. Cut them into sizes that fit your juicer's chute.
3. Juice the kale, cucumber, green apples, lemon, ginger, and mint leaves.
4. Stir well and pour into a glass. Experience the cleansing power of this green citrus juice.

Refreshing Zesty Green Fusion:

Ingredients

- 3 cups spinach leaves
- green bell pepper, seeds removed
- celery stalks
- lime
- green pear
- parsley

Directions:

1. Wash all the ingredients thoroughly.
2. Cut them into sizes that fit your juicer's chute.
3. Juice the spinach, green bell pepper, celery, lime, pear, parsley.

4. Mix well and pour into a glass. Enjoy the refreshing and detoxifying benefits of this green detox juice. These green juice recipes are packed with detoxifying ingredients that support your body's natural cleansing processes. Incorporate them into your routine to revitalize your body and promote a sense of well-being. Stay tuned for more juicing inspiration and tips tomorrow!

Day 10: Adding Superfoods to Your Green Juices

Welcome to day 10! Today, let us explore the world of superfoods and how you can elevate your green juices to a whole new level by incorporating these nutrient-packed ingredients. Superfoods offer a wide range of health benefits. Here are two green juice recipes featuring powerful superfoods:

Kale & Spirulina Energizer:

Ingredients
- 2 cups kale leaves
- 1 cucumber
- 1 green apple
- 1 lemon
- 1-inch piece of ginger
- 1 teaspoon spirulina powder

Directions:
1. Wash all the ingredients thoroughly.
2. Cut them into sizes that fit your juicer's chute.
3. Juice the kale, cucumber, green apple, lemon, and ginger.
4. Stir in the spirulina powder until well combined.
5. Pour it into a glass and enjoy this energizing kale and spirulina juice.

Spinach & Chia Seed Vitality Booster:
Ingredients
- 3 cups spinach leaves
- celery stalk
- pear
- lime
- tablespoon chia seeds
- 1-2 teaspoons honey or agave syrup (optional for sweetness)

Directions:
1. Wash all the ingredients thoroughly.
2. Cut them into sizes that fit your juicer's chute.
3. Juice the spinach, celery, pear, and lime.
4. Put your chia seeds in your juice and let them sit for 5-10 minutes to allow the chia seeds to absorb liquid.
5. Add honey or agave syrup if desired for a touch of sweetness.
6. Mix well and pour into a glass. Experience the vitality-boosting goodness of this spinach and chia seed juice.

By adding superfoods like spirulina and chia seeds to your green juices, you enhance their nutritional content and create drinks that nourish your body and mind. Stay tuned for more juicing inspiration and valuable tips tomorrow!

Happy juicing! □□□

Day 11: Juicing for Weight Loss
Welcome to Day 11! Today, let us focus on how cold press juicing can help you in your weight loss journey.
Juicing for weight loss is not about extreme diets but rather incorporating nutrient-dense, low-calorie juices into your daily routine. Here are some tips and a refreshing weight loss juice recipe to support your goals:

Tips for Juicing for Weight Loss:

1. **Make sure to focus on Vegetables:** Since vegetables can be low in calories and high in fiber, it makes them ideal for weight loss. Incorporate a variety of greens like spinach, kale, and celery into your juices.
2. **Moderate Fruit Intake:** While fruits are healthy, they also contain natural sugars. opt for low-sugar fruits like berries and apples and use them in moderation to control your calorie intake.
3. **Include Protein:** Adding a source of protein to your juices, such as chia seeds, hemp seeds, or a scoop of plant-based protein powder can help you feel fuller for longer, reducing overall calorie consumption.

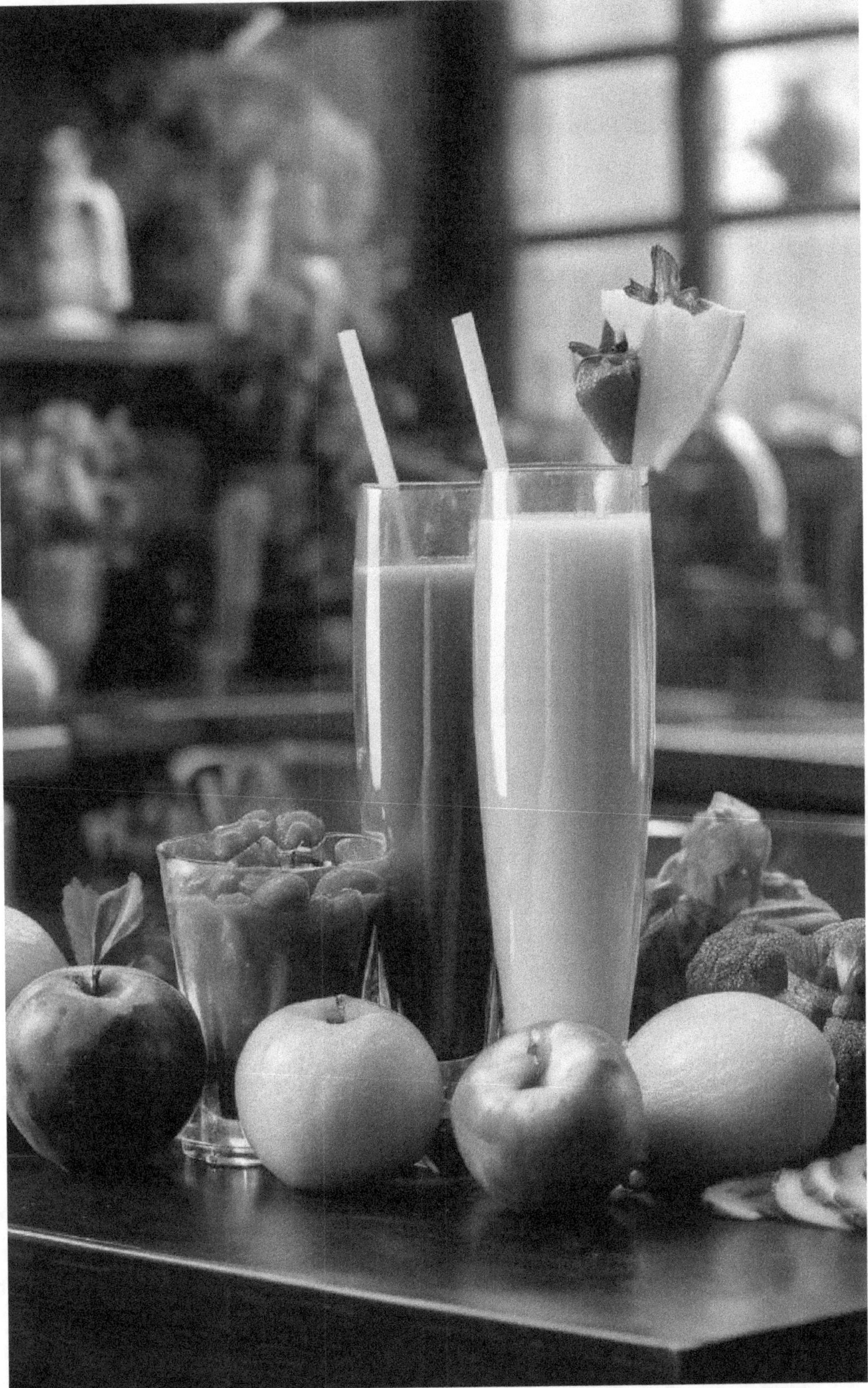

4. **Stay Hydrated:** Proper hydration is essential for weight loss. Use hydrating ingredients like cucumber and watermelon in your juices to keep your body well hydrated.

5. **Mindful Drinking:** Pay attention to portion sizes.
Even though juices are healthy, consuming them in excess can lead to excess calorie intake. Stick to moderate portions.

Weight Loss Juice Recipe:

Green Slimming Elixir

Ingredients:

- 2 cups spinach
- cucumber
- green apple
- 1/2 lemon
- 1-inch piece of ginger
- tablespoon chia seeds

Directions:

1. Wash all the ingredients thoroughly.
2. Cut them into sizes that fit your juicer's chute.
3. Juice the spinach, cucumber, green apple, lemon, and ginger.
4. Stir in the chia seeds and let the mixture sit for 5-10 minutes to allow the chia seeds to absorb liquid.
5. Mix well and pour into a glass. Savor the refreshing taste of this Green Slimming Elixir, designed to support your weight loss goals.

By incorporating nutrient-packed, low-calorie juices, you will be boosting your metabolism and increasing your energy levels and aid your weight loss journey in a healthy way. Stay tuned for more juicing tips and delicious recipes tomorrow!

Happy juicing! □□□

Day 12: DIY Juice Cleanses at Home

Welcome to Day 12! Today, let's explore the concept of juice cleansing and how you can create your DIY juice cleansers at home. Juice cleansers are short-term diets that involve consuming only fresh juices from fruits and vegetables. They are believed to detoxify, boost your energy, and promote overall well-being. Here is how you can design your one-day juice cleanse:

Morning Juice: Citrus Wake-Up Call

Ingredients

- 3 oranges (peeled)
- grapefruit (peeled)
- lemon (peeled)
- 1-inch piece of ginger

Directions:

1. Juice the oranges, grapefruit, lemon, and ginger.
2. Mix well and start your day with this refreshing citrus wake-up call juice.

Mid-Morning Juice: Green Revitalizer

Ingredients:

- 2 cups spinach leaves
- cucumber
- green apples

- 1/2 lime
- tablespoon chia seeds

Directions:

1. Juice the spinach, cucumber, green apples, and lime.
2. Stir in the chia seeds and let it sit for 5-10 minutes so that chia seeds can absorb the liquid.
3. Mix well and enjoy this green revitalizer juice for a midmorning boost.

Lunchtime Juice: Veggie Vitality

Ingredients

- 3 carrots
- red beetroot
- celery stalk
- 1/2 lemon (peeled)
- 1-inch piece of turmeric piece of ginger

Directions

1. Juice the carrots, beetroot, celery, lemon, ginger, and turmeric.
2. Pour into a glass and enjoy the nutrients of this veggie vitality juice for your lunch.

Afternoon Snack: Berry Bliss

Ingredients

- lemon
- 1/2 cup blueberries
- 1/2 cup coconut water
- honey or agave syrup (optional)

Directions:
1. Juice the blueberries and lemon
2. Mix in the coconut water and add honey or agave syrup
3. Enjoy your delightful berry bliss juice. Drink plenty of water throughout the day to stay hydrated during your juice cleansing. While short-term juicing can be beneficial, you must consult your healthcare professional before making significant changes to your diet. Stay tuned for more juicing tips and exciting recipes tomorrow!
Happy juicing! □□□

Day 13: Juicing for Glowing Skin

Welcome to Day 13! Today, let us explore how the right combination of fruits and vegetables in your juices can promote radiant and glowing skin. Clear, healthy skin often starts from within, and juicing can help your skin with the essential nutrients it needs to look its best.

Here are some skin-loving ingredients and a rejuvenating Juice recipe to enhance your skin's natural glow.

Skin-Loving Ingredients

1. Vitamin C: Found in citrus fruits like oranges, lemons, and grapefruits, vitamin C is crucial for collagen production, which maintains skin elasticity and prevents signs of aging.
2. Beta-Carotene: Carrots, sweet potatoes, and kale are rich in beta-carotene, a precursor to vitamin A. Vitamin A promotes skin cell turnover and helps maintain a healthy complexion.

3. Antioxidants: Berries like blueberries, strawberries, and raspberries are loaded with antioxidants, which protect the skin from free radical damage and support a youthful appearance.

4. Hydration: Cucumbers and watermelons have high water content, keeping your skin hydrated and preventing dryness and flakiness.

Rejuvenating Skin Glow Juice:

Ingredients

- 2 oranges (peeled)
- 1/2 cucumber
- carrot (peeled)
- Handful of strawberries
- 1/2 lemon (peeled)
- 1-inch piece of ginger
- tablespoon flaxseeds (for omega-3 fatty acids and skin health)

Directions:

1. Juice oranges, cucumber, carrot, strawberries, lemon, and ginger.

2. Stir in the flaxseeds for an extra boost of skin nourishing omega-3 fatty acids.

3. Pour into a glass and relish the rejuvenating effects of this skin glow juice. Incorporating these skin-loving ingredients into your juices, you provide your skin with essential vitamins, minerals, and antioxidants to maintain a healthy, radiant glow.

Stay tuned for more juicing tips and delightful recipes tomorrow!

Happy juicing! □□□□

Day 14: Juicing for Mental Clarity and Focus

Welcome to day 14! Today, let us explore the connection between the nutrients in fresh juices and mental clarity. Certain fruits and vegetables are known for their brain- boosting properties, helping enhance focus, concentration, and overall cognitive function. Here are some ingredients and a revitalizing juice recipe to support mental clarity and focus:

Brain-Boosting Ingredients:

1. **Blueberries:** Packed with antioxidants, blueberries are known to improve memory and cognitive performance. They also help protect the brain from oxidative stress.

2. **Spinach and kale:** are rich in vitamins A and K, folate, and iron, promoting healthy brain function and helps with mental clarity.

3. **Turmeric:** Curcumin, the active compound in turmeric, has anti-inflammatory and antioxidant properties that support brain health and may help prevent neurodegenerative diseases.

4. **Omega-3 Fatty Acids:** Flaxseeds are a major source of alpha-linolenic acid (ALA), a type of omega-3 fatty acid.

Omega-3s support brain structure and aid in neurotransmitter function, promoting mental focus.

Revitalizing Brain-Boosting Juice:

Ingredients

1 cup blueberries

2 cups spinach leaves

1 cucumber

1 orange (peeled)

1-inch piece of turmeric

1 tablespoon flaxseeds (ground for better absorption)

Directions:
1. Wash all the ingredients thoroughly.
2. Cut them into sizes that fit your juicer's chute.
3. Juice the blueberries, spinach, cucumber, orange, and turmeric.
4. Stir in the ground flaxseeds for an extra dose of brain- boosting omega-3s.
5. Pour it into a glass and enjoy this revitalizing juice to enhance your mental clarity and focus.

 Embrace the power of green juices in your daily routine.
Their vibrant flavors and health-boosting properties make them a wonderful addition to your juicing repertoire. Stay tuned for more juicing tips and exciting recipes tomorrow!

Happy juicing! □ □ □

By incorporating these brain-boosting ingredients into your juices, you are nourishing your brain and supporting cognitive function. Regular consumption of nutrient-dense juices can contribute to improved mental clarity, focus, and overall brain health. Stay tuned for more juicing insights and exciting recipes tomorrow!

Day 15: Celebrating Your Juicing Journey
Congratulations on reaching Day 15 of your cold press juicing adventure! Today, it is time to celebrate your dedication to nourishing your body, mind, and soul with fresh, vibrant juices. As you reflect on the past two weeks, remember the progress you have made, the delicious recipes you have tried, and the positive impact juicing has had on your overall well-being. Take a Moment to Reflect:

1. **Acknowledge Your Achievements:** Whether you started juicing for health, weight loss, or simply to incorporate more fruits and vegetables into your diet, acknowledge the progress that you have made so far. Celebrate the steps you've taken towards a healthier lifestyle.

2. **Embrace the Journey:** Juicing is not just a temporary diet but a lifestyle choice. Embrace this journey you have embarked upon and continue to explore new recipes, flavors, and ingredients. The world of juicing is full of endless possibilities.

3. **Always listen to Your Body:** Pay attention to how your body feels after incorporating fresh juices into your diet. Notice any changes in your energy levels, skin, digestion, or overall mood. Your body has its way of telling you what it needs.

Celebrate with a Special Juice:

The Jubilant Drink

Ingredients

- red beetroot
- red apple
- carrots
- orange
- 1-inch piece of ginger
- Handful of fresh mint leaves
- Splash of coconut water

Directions:

1. Wash all the ingredients thoroughly.
2. Cut them into sizes that fit your juicer's chute.
3. Juice the beetroot, carrots, orange, ginger, and mint leaves.
4. Add your splash of coconut water and stir well.
5. Pour it into a glass and raise it to your successful juicing journey!

Continue the Juicing Adventure: As you celebrate your achievements today, remember that your juicing journey does not have to end here. Keep exploring new flavors, experimenting with different ingredients, and enjoying the multitude of health benefits that fresh juices offer. Stay tuned for more juicing tips, recipes, and inspiration in the days to come. Cheers to your health and vitality!

Happy juicing!

Day 16: Post-Juicing Transition and Maintenance
Welcome to Day 16, the first day after completing your 15-day cold press juicing journey! Congratulations on your dedication and commitment to your health. As you go back to your regular diet, it is important to do so mindfully by remembering the benefits you have learned. Here are a few ideas to help you smoothly transition and maintain your well-being:

1. **Gradual Reintroduction:** Slowly reintroduce solid foods into your diet, starting with easily digestible fruits, vegetables, and whole grains. Avoid heavy and processed foods initially.

2. **Portion Control:** Pay attention to your portion sizes and listen to your body's hunger and fullness cues. Juicing may have reset your appetite, so pay attention to how much you are eating.

3. **Hydration:** Continue to prioritize hydration. Water, herbal teas, and infused water with fresh fruits and herbs are excellent choices to stay hydrated.

4. **Balanced Diet:** Focus on a balanced diet that includes a variety of fruits, vegetables, whole grains, lean proteins, and healthy fats. This diverse diet provides essential nutrients for overall health.

5. **Mindful Eating:** Practice mindful eating by being present during meals. Chew and enjoy your food thoroughly and savor the flavors. Avoid distractions like TV or smartphones while eating.

6. **Regular Exercise:** Make sure you have regular physical activity in your daily routine. Exercising not only supports your physical health but also enhances your mental wellbeing.

7. **Post-Juicing Recipes:** Consider incorporating juices into your routine as meal replacements or snacks. For example, a green smoothie with peanut butter, spinach, banana, almond milk, and a scoop of protein powder can be a satisfying and nutritious option.

8. **Reflect and Set Goals:** Take a moment to reflect on your juicing journey. Consider what worked well for you and set achievable health goals for the future, whether it's incorporating more vegetables into your meals or practicing mindfulness.

Remember, your juicing journey was a positive step towards a healthier lifestyle. Use the knowledge and habits you've gained to continue making nourishing choices for your body. Stay tuned for more health and wellness tips in the days ahead. Wishing you continued health and vitality! □□□

Day 17: Embracing Long-Term Health Habits

Welcome to Day 17, where we delve into the importance of embracing long-term health habits after completing your 15-day cold press juicing journey. You have laid a solid foundation for a healthier lifestyle, and now it's time to focus on building on it. You can use these strategies to help you maintain your health and vitality in the long run:

1. **Whole Foods Diet:** Focus on consuming whole foods that are not processed. Eat a colorful variety of fruits, vegetables, whole grains, lean proteins, and healthy fats in your meals. These nutrient-dense foods can provide essential vitamins, minerals, and antioxidants.

2. **Mindful Eating:** Constantly be mindful of your eating by being aware of your food choices and eating habits. Listen to your body's

hunger and fullness cues and savor each bite. Avoid emotional or distracted eating.

3. **Regular Exercise:** You will need to have some type of physical routine as part of your day. Try for at least 60 minutes of moderate to-intensity exercising or 30 minutes of vigorous to-intensity exercising per day. Also, incorporate some type of muscle training activities on two or more days a week.

4. **Getting enough sleep:** should be a priority 7-9 hours of sound sleep each night. Sound sleep is essential for your overall health, mood regulation, and for everyday function.

5. **Stress Managing:** Find ways to manage your stress, such as walking, reading, listening to music, or hobbies that you enjoy doing. Chronic stress can negatively impact your health, so it's important to find healthy coping mechanisms.

6. **Hydration:** throughout the day drink plenty of water. Being hydrated supports your digestive system, metabolism, and your complete well-being.

7. **Health Checkups:** Regular checkups with your healthcare provider are key as well. Regular screenings and health assessments can help detect potential issues early, allowing for timely interventions.

8. **Healthy Relationships:** Cultivate positive, supportive relationships with friends and family. Social connections and a dedicated support system contribute to emotional well-being.

9. **Stay Curious:** Keep learning about nutrition, fitness, and overall wellness. Stay curious and open-minded about innovative approaches to health, allowing yourself to evolve and adapt.

Integrating these long-term health habits into your daily life, you will continue to nurture your well-being and enjoy a better quality of life. Staying committed to your healthy journey will help with improving your health over time, and you will reap the benefits for years to come. Wishing you continued health and happiness on your path to wellness! □□□

Day 18: Cultivating a Positive Mindset

Welcome to Day 18, where we focus on the power of a positive mindset in achieving and maintaining a healthy life. Having a positive mental attitude plays a crucial role in your overall well-being. Cultivating a positive mindset can enhance your motivation, resilience, and overall happiness. Here are some strategies to help you foster a positive outlook on this journey:

1. **Having Gratitude:** Reflect for a few moments each morning to reflect on what you're grateful for. Gratitude can shift your focus from what you lack to what you have, fostering positivity and contentment with health and positivity!

2. **Affirmations:** Use positive affirmations to challenge and control negative thoughts. Repeat affirmations related to your health and well-being to reinforce positive beliefs about yourself.

3. **Visualize Success:** Visualize yourself achieving your health goals. Imagine the feeling of accomplishment and the positive changes in your life. Visualization can boost your confidence and motivation.

4. **Surround Yourself with Positivity:** Spend time with people who uplift and have been there for you. You will want to have positive

social interactions because it can have a significant impact on your mood and mindset.

5. **Learn from Challenges:** Instead of viewing setbacks as failures, see them as opportunities to gain experience and grow. Embrace challenges as a chance to develop resilience and critical thinking skills.

6. **Mindful Breathing:** Practice mindful breathing exercises to calm your mind and reduce stress. Deep, intentional breathing can bring clarity and focus to your thoughts.

7. **Avoid Comparison:** Do not compare your life or progress to anybody else. Your journey is unique for you. Focus on your accomplishments and celebrate your small and big milestones.

8. **Self-Compassion:** Be kind to yourself. Care for and love yourself the same way you love and care for a close friend. Show yourself kindness and compassion, especially during difficult times.

9. **Acknowledge your Small Wins:** Celebrate your achievements, no matter how small they may seem. Every step forward is a victory worth celebrating.

Having a positive mindset can help you navigate challenging times more effectively can help you stay motivated and maintain your commitment to a healthy lifestyle. Remember, your thoughts have a powerful influence on your actions and outcomes. Stay positive, stay focused, and keep moving forward on your journey to well-being.

Wishing you continued positivity and success on your health and happiness journey! □□

Day 19: Embracing Self-Care Habits

Welcome to Day 19! Today, let us focus on the importance of self-care and how it contributes to your overall wellbeing. Self-care is not selfish; it's a vital practice that allows you to take care of your physical needs, and have a healthy mental state, as well as your emotional health.

Below you will find some self-care habits to consider adopting into your routine:

1. **Sleep:** Create a relaxing bedtime ritual that will help you get quality sleep for at least 7 to 9 hours and have a comfortable sleeping environment and prioritize sleep as a non-negotiable part of your day.

2. **Nourish Your Body:** Be mindful of your nutritional needs. try to eat a balanced diet of fruits, vegetables, whole grains, lean proteins, and healthy fats. Hydrating your body with water, herbal teas, and infused water with fresh fruits and herbs is another way to drink water.

3. **Keep it Moving Your Body:** With activities you enjoy. Whether it's walking, dancing, yoga, or any other form of exercise, regular movement not only supports your physical health but also boosts your mood and energy levels.

4. **Practice Mindfulness:** Incorporate mindfulness practices such as sitting still, praying, or journaling. These practices can help reduce stress, increase self-awareness, and enhance your overall sense of well-being.

5. **Set Boundaries:** Learn to say no to commitments or activities that drain your energy or cause stress. Set healthy boundaries to protect your time and mental space.

6. **Hobbies:** Learn and do activities that bring you joy and relaxation. Whether it is painting, gardening, doing crafts, or any other hobby, dedicating time to activities you love can be incredibly rejuvenating.

7. **Connect with Loved Ones:** Maintain meaningful connections with family and friends. Spending quality time with loved ones and nurturing relationships provides emotional support and a sense of belonging.

8. **Unplug:** Take breaks from screens, social media, and news. Constant exposure to digital devices can contribute to stress and overwhelm. Allocate specific times in your day for unplugging from technology.

9. **Seeking Professional help:** Do not hesitate to seek support from mental health professionals if you're feeling overwhelmed, anxious, or stressed. Therapy or counseling can provide valuable tools and coping strategies.

Remember, self-care looks different for everyone. It is about identifying what brings you peace, joy, and relaxation.

By embracing self-care habits, you invest in your overall well-being and create a solid foundation for a healthier, happier you. Take a moment today to engage in a self-care activity that resonates with you.

You deserve it! □□

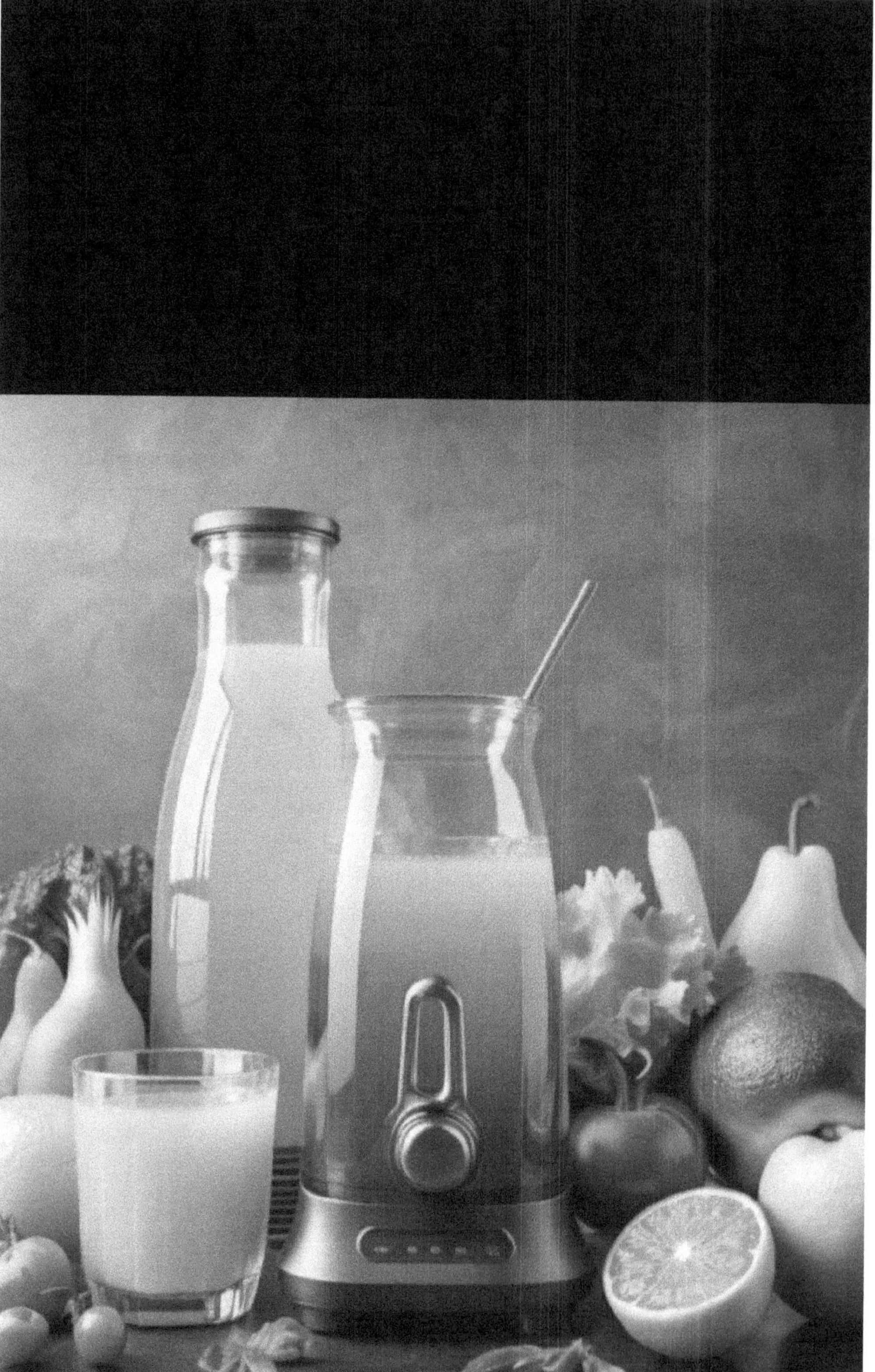

Day 20: Reflecting on Your Wellness Journey

Welcome to Day 20, a significant milestone in your wellness journey! Today, take some time to reflect on the progress you have made, the lessons you have learned, and the positive changes you have experienced. Reflecting on your journey can provide valuable insights and motivation to continue your path to well-being.

Here are some prompts to guide your reflection:

1. **Celebrating Achievements:** Take note of your achievements, both big and small. Celebrate your successes, whether it is incorporating more fruits and vegetables into your diet, improving your fitness level, or adopting healthier habits.

2. **Challenges and Learnings:** Reflect on the challenges you faced and the lessons you learned from them.

Challenges are opportunities for growth and learning. What insights have you gained from overcoming obstacles?

3. **Mind-Body Connection:** Consider the connection between your mental and physical well-being. How has your mental outlook influenced your physical health, and vice versa? Have you noticed changes in your mood, energy levels, or overall mindset?

4. **Gratitude:** Practice gratitude for the positive aspects of your journey. What are you grateful for in your life right now? Cultivating gratitude can enhance your overall sense of contentment and happiness.

5. **Future Goals:** Set realistic and achievable goals for your continued wellness journey. What do you hope to accomplish in the coming

weeks and months? Setting specific goals can provide direction and motivation.

6. **Self-Compassion:** Reflect on your relationship with yourself. Have you been kind and compassionate toward yourself during this journey? Self-compassion is a powerful tool for personal growth and well-being.

7. **Support:** Acknowledge and surround yourself with people who can support and who can significantly impact your motivation and success.

8. **Self-Discovery:** Consider any new things you have discovered about yourself during this journey. What activities bring you joy? What coping strategies work best for managing stress? Self-discovery is an ongoing process that enriches your life.

Take this time to appreciate your efforts and the positive changes you have made. Your commitment to your health and well-being is inspiring. As you continue your journey, remember that every step forward is a victory.

Stay motivated, stay positive, and keep nurturing your mind, body, and soul. I Wish you continued success and fulfillment on your wellness path! □□

Day 21: Embracing Sustainable Wellness

Congratulations on reaching Day 21, marking the completion of your three-week wellness journey! As you reflect on the last three weeks and all the positive changes you have made, it is essential to focus on maintaining these healthy habits overall. Sustainable wellness is about integrating positive lifestyle changes into your daily routine. Here are some key principles to help you embrace sustainable wellness:

1. **Consistency over Perfection:** Aim for consistency rather than perfection. Small, consistent efforts over time lead significant improvements. It is okay to have occasional setbacks; what is most important is your commitment and ability to get back on track.

2. **Listen to Your Body:** Pay attention to your body's signals. Rest when you need it, nourish yourself with healthy foods and engage in physical activity that feels good. Your body knows best what it needs.

3. **Flexibility and Adaptability:** Be flexible with your routines. Life can be unpredictable, and circumstances change. Learn to adapt your wellness practices to different situations without feeling discouraged.

4. **Mindful Eating:** Continue to be aware and mindful of your eating. Savor each bite and listen to your body's hunger and fullness cues. Avoid emotional eating and eat with intention.

Day 22: Cultivating Positive Habits

Welcome to Day 22! Today, let us look at cultivating positive habits that contribute to your overall well-being. Habits are powerful—they shape your daily routine, influence your choices, and define your lifestyle.

By cultivating positive habits, you can have a healthier and fulfilling life. Here are some habits to consider incorporating into your routine:

1. **Morning Routine:** Establish a positive morning routine that sets the tone for your day. This could include activities like stretching, meditating, journaling, or enjoying a healthy breakfast. A mindful

morning routine can help with your mood and energy levels for that day.

2. **Hydration Habit:** Carry a reusable water bottle with you to stay hydrated, aiding digestion, supporting skin health, and maintaining overall bodily functions.

3. **Nutritious Choices:** Make nutritious food choices. To avoid impulsive eating plan your meals ahead of time.

4. Physical Activity: Whether it's a morning workout, a walk during your lunch break or an evening yoga session, find activities you enjoy staying active and energized.

5. **Gratitude Practice:** As we mention earlier, create a gratitude habit for a few minutes each day to think about the things you are grateful for. Gratitude can shift your perspective and enhance your peace and your overall happiness.

6. **Digital Detox:** Dedicate time in your day to unplug for a digital detox. Especially before bedtime, to improve sleep quality and reduce stress.

7. **Evening Wind-Down:** Create a calming evening routine to help you unwind and prepare for a restful night's sleep.
This could include reading, taking a warm bath, practicing relaxation exercises, or meditating.

8. **Connect with and to Nature:** Find some time to be outdoors to connect with your outside surroundings. You can run, walk, or sit in the park, planting, or tiling gardening, or simply sitting in a natural Being in nature can reduce stress and boost your mood.

By incorporating these positive habits into your daily life, you are investing in your physical, mental, and emotional well-being. Remember, habits are formed through consistency and repetition, so be patient with yourself as you cultivate these positive changes. Stay committed, stay positive, and enjoy the journey of creating a healthier, happier you! □□□

Day 23: Practicing Mindfulness

Welcome to Day 23 of your wellness journey! Today, let us explore the practice of mindfulness. Mindfulness involves being fully present and aware of the current moment, without judgment to yourself or anybody else. Practicing mindfulness can help with reducing your stress levels, improve your focus, and give you a greater sense of calmness and contentment.

1. **Mindful Breathing:** find a few minutes in your day to focus on your breath. Inhale slowly through your nose, fill your lungs with air then breathe out gently. Notice the sensation of your breath.

2. **Do a scan of your body:** Find a peaceful place to sit or lie down. Bring your attention to different various parts of your body by closing your eyes, starting from your feet, and moving up to your head. Notice any sensations, tension, or relaxation in each area. This practice promotes body awareness.

3. **Mindful Eating**: During your next meal, pay attention to the flavors, textures, and smells of your food. Chew your food thoroughly and be

present with each mouthful. Mindful eating can enhance your enjoyment of food and help prevent overeating.

   4. **Nature Observation:** Spend time outdoors and observe nature mindfully. Notice the colors, shapes, and movements of the natural world around you. Listen to the sounds of birds chirping or leaves rustling in the wind. Engage your senses in nature.

   5. **Thankful Journaling:** Write down three things you are grateful for today. It could be that you are grateful for life, health, moments of kindness, or positive aspects of your life.
Regular gratitude journaling can shift your focus toward positivity and enhance your overall well-being.

6. **Mindful Walking:** Go for a walk and when you do be mindful of each step you take. Pay attention to the ground beneath your feet, notice the rhythm of your steps, and be aware of your surroundings. Walking mindfully can be a calming and grounding experience.

7. **Mindful Pause:** Throughout your day, take short mindful pauses. Stop whatever you're doing, take a few deep breaths, and bring your awareness to the present moment. This practice can help you reset and approach your tasks with renewed focus.

8. **Mindfulness:** is a skill that can be developed with practice, so be patient with yourself as you explore these techniques. Enjoy the peace and mindfulness that this practice brings to your life! ⬜⬜

Day 24: Cultivating Compassion

Welcome to Day 24 of your wellness journey! Today, let us focus on cultivating compassion, both for others and for yourself. Compassion is the ability to empathize with the suffering of others and the desire to alleviate that suffering. When you practice compassion, you create a positive impact not only on others but also on your wellbeing. Here are some ways to cultivate compassion in your life:

1. **Random Acts of Kindness:** Perform random acts of kindness throughout your day. It could be as simple as offering a genuine compliment, holding the door open for someone, or helping a friend or colleague in need. Acts of kindness create a ripple effect of positivity.

2. **Active Listening:** Practice active listening when interacting with others. Give your full attention, maintain eye contact, and show empathy. By truly listening, you are letting the person know that you value their feelings.

3. **Self-Compassion:** Be kind to others, forgive and have compassion. Treat yourself with the same warmth and care that you would offer to others.

4. **Volunteer or Help Others:** Engage in volunteer work or help those in need. Volunteering your time or skills to support a cause or assist others can foster a deep sense of compassion and fulfillment.

5. **Express Gratitude:** Express gratitude to and for people in your life who have made a positive impact. Write a heartfelt note, make a phone call, or simply express your gratitude in person. Showing appreciation fosters connections and deepens relationships.

6. **Forgiveness:** Practice forgiveness, both for others and for yourself. Holding onto grudges or self-blame can cause emotional distress. Letting go and forgiving can free you from negativity and promote emotional healing.

7. **Empathy Practice:** Put yourself in someone else's shoes and try to understand their perspective, feelings, and experiences. Developing empathy allows you to connect with others on a deeper level and respond with compassion.

8. **Mindful Compassion Meditation:** Engage compassion meditation practice. Focus on your breath, and see yourself sending feelings of love, compassion, and well- being to yourself and others. This practice can enhance your sense of connection and compassion.

By cultivating compassion in your daily life, you contribute to a more compassionate and empathetic world. Compassion not only benefits others but also enriches your own life, fostering a sense of purpose and fulfillment. Embrace the power of compassion, and let it guide your interactions and relationships. Wishing you a day filled with kindness and warmth! □□

Day 25: Embracing Hope

Welcome to Day 25! Today, let us explore the concept of hope and how it can give you the power to overcome objections and bounce back from defeat. Hope is the ability to adapt and recover from tricky situations, defeats, or hardships. Pursuing hope can enhance your mental and emotional well-being. Here are some ways to embrace resilience in your life:

1. **Positive Mindset:** Maintain a positive outlook, even in challenging situations. Focus on what you can control and look for opportunities for growth and learning in every experience. A positive mindset can help you navigate difficulties with grace and determination.

2. **Critical Thinking Skills:** Develop effective problem-solving skills. Break challenges into smaller, manageable steps and consider different solutions. Seek support and advice when needed. Building your critical thinking skills enhances your ability to face challenges confidently.

3. **Self-Compassion:** Be gentle with yourself during tough times. Treat yourself with kindness and understanding.

Acknowledge your feelings without judgment and remind yourself that setbacks are a natural part of life. Self-compassion strengthens your emotional resilience.

4. **Healthy Coping Strategies:** Cultivate healthy coping strategies to manage stress and your emotions. Learn some techniques that can relax you, journal your thoughts regularly, or seek support from your family and friends or a professional counselor. Healthy coping mechanisms can build your resilience and hope.

5. **Maintain Supportive Relationships:** Surround yourself with supportive and positive people. Maintain strong connections with friends, family, or support groups. Having a reliable support system can provide emotional strength during challenging times.

6. **Acceptance of Change:** Embrace change as a natural part of life. Life is constantly evolving, and resilience lies in adapting to new

circumstances. Embrace change with an open mind and view it as an opportunity for personal growth and transformation.

7. **Practice appreciation:** Practice appreciation even in tough times. Reflect on the things you are grateful for, no matter how small.

8. **Gratitude:** fosters a positive outlook and resilience by focusing on the positive aspects of your life.

9. **Learn from Setbacks:** View setbacks as opportunities for learning and growth. Reflect on the lessons you have gained from past challenges. Every setback can offer valuable insights and resilience-building experiences.

By embracing resilience, you strengthen your ability to face life's challenges with courage and grace. Remember those setbacks do not define you; your response to them does. Embrace your inner strength, stay positive, and keep moving forward with confidence. You are more resilient than you realize.

Wishing you a day filled with resilience and strength! □□

Day 26: Cultivating Mindful Habits

Welcome to Day 26! Today, let us explore the practice of acquiring mindful habits, which can greatly increase your overall well-being. Mindful habits involve being deliberate in your actions, thoughts, and choices. By Integrating mindfulness into your daily routines, can reduce stress, improve focus, and deepen your sense of contentment. Here are some mindful habits to consider integrating into your life:

1. **Mindful Breathing:** Begin your day with Mindful breathing because it can help you center yourself and set the tone for the day.
2. **Mindful Eating:** Pay attention to the details of the colors, textures, and flavors of your food. Chew your food slowly, savoring each bite. Be present with your meal, appreciating the nourishment it provides.
3. **Digital Mindfulness:** Be mindful of your screen time. Designated periods for using your devices and practice unplugging during meals and before bedtime. Mindful technology use can improve your focus and promote better sleep.
4. **Mindful Walking:** Take a walk outdoors. Be aware of the sensation of your feet touching the ground, the sounds of nature, and the movement of your body. Walking mindfully can be a meditative experience, grounding you in the present moment.
5. **Take a few minutes:** to reflect on three things you are grateful for each day. Writing them down in a gratitude journal can deepen your sense of appreciation and positivity.
6. **Mindful Communication:** Practice active listening during phone calls and conversations with others. Pay close attention and keep eye contact and give your complete attention to the person speaking. Mindful communication strengthens your connections with others.
7. **Mindful Reflection:** Dedicate a few minutes each evening to reflect on your day. Acknowledge your achievements, express gratitude for positive moments, and consider areas where you can grow. Mindful reflection promotes self-awareness and personal growth.

8. **Mindful Pause:** Take mindful pauses throughout your day. Stop whatever you are doing, take a few deep breaths, and bring your awareness to the present moment. Mindful pauses can reset your focus and reduce stress.

By cultivating these mindful habits, you invite greater awareness and presence into your daily life. Mindfulness allows you to experience each moment fully and respond to life's challenges with clarity and calmness. Embrace the practice of mindfulness, and you'll find greater peace and fulfillment in your journey.
Wishing you a day filled with mindful moments! □□

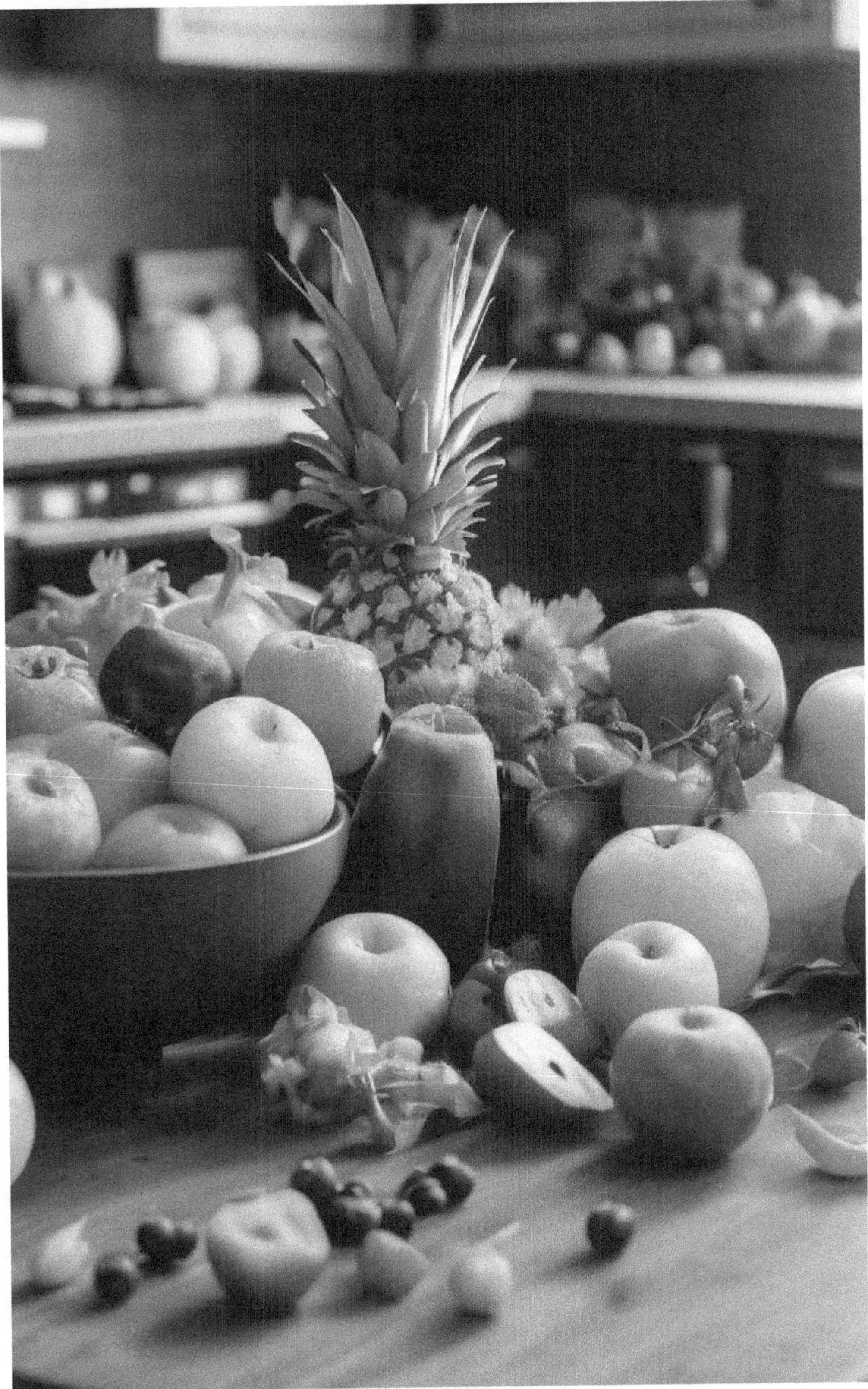

Day 27: Practicing Self-Reflection

Welcome to Day 27! Today, let us focus on the powerful practice of self-reflection. Self-reflection involves taking the time to contemplate your thoughts, feelings, and experiences. It is a valuable tool for personal growth, self- awareness, and gaining insights into your life. Here are some ways to practice self-reflection:

1. **Journaling:** Set aside time to write in a journal. Reflect on your day, your emotions, and any challenges you face or have faced. Write about your achievements, no matter how small, and express gratitude for positive experiences. Journaling provides clarity and helps you process your thoughts.

2. **Guided Reflection:** Use guided reflection exercises or prompts to delve deeper into your thoughts and feelings.

There are various resources, such as books, apps, and online platforms, which offer guided reflection exercises tailored to several aspects of your life.

3. **Mindful Meditation:** Practice mindful meditation with focus on self-reflection. Sit in a quiet space, close your eyes, and bring your attention inward. Reflect on your thoughts and emotions without judgment.

4. **Life Assessment:** Think about different parts of your life, such as relationships, career, health, and personal development. Ask yourself what is going well in each area and where you would like to see improvement. Identifying areas for growth can guide your future actions.

5. **Past Experiences:** Reflect on past experiences and lessons you have learned from them. Consider how these experiences have shaped your beliefs, values, and behaviors. Understanding your past can give and knowledge and clarity about your present self.

6. **Goals and Aspirations:** Reflect on your goals, both short-term and long-term. Evaluate your progress and consider whether your goals are still aligned with your values and aspirations. Adjust your goals if necessary, keeping them in harmony with your evolving self.

7. **Self-Compassion:** Practice self-compassion during yourself-reflection. Be kind and understanding toward yourself, acknowledging your strengths and areas for improvement. Treat yourself with the same love and encouragement you would offer a dear friend.

8. **Gratitude for Growth:** Express gratitude for your growth journey. Acknowledge the progress you have made, the challenges you've overcome, and the person you have become. Gratitude for your growth fuels your motivation to continue evolving.

By engaging in self-reflection, you gain a deeper understanding of yourself, your goals, and your desires. It empowers you to make conscious choices, align your actions with your values, and continue your journey toward a fulfilling life. Embrace the practice of self-reflection, and you will find valuable insights and clarity on your path to personal growth.

Wishing you a day filled with meaningful self-discovery!

 □□

Day 28: Cultivating Gratitude

Welcome to Day 28! Today, let us explore the transformative power of gratitude. Cultivating gratitude involves recognizing and appreciating the positive aspects of your life, both big and small.

Practicing gratitude regularly can enhance your overall well-being, boost your mood, and increase your life satisfaction.

1. **Gratitude Journal:** Dedicate a few minutes each day to writing down three things which you are grateful for. They can be simple pleasures, moments of kindness, or aspects of your life that bring you joy. Keeping a gratitude journal helps you focus on the positive aspects of your day.

2. **Gratitude Jar:** Create a gratitude jar and place it in a visible location. Whenever you experience something, you are grateful for, write it on a small piece of paper and place it in the jar. Over time, the jar will fill with reminders of the good things in your life.

3. **Express Gratitude:** Take the time to express your gratitude to others. Write a heartfelt thank-you note, send a message of appreciation, or simply verbalize your gratitude in person. Expressing gratitude strengthens your relationships and spreads positivity.

4. **Morning Gratitude Practice:** Start your day with gratitude practice. Before getting out of bed, think of three things you are grateful for. It could be the warmth of the sun, the breath in your body, the support of your loved ones, or the opportunities the day holds.

5. **Setting a positive tone:** in the morning can influence your entire day.

6. **Gratitude Walk:** Take a gratitude walk outdoors. As you walk, focus on the things you're grateful for in nature—the sound of birds, the beauty of flowers, or the warmth of the sun. Engaging your senses in gratitude amplifies your appreciation for the world around you.

7. **Gratitude Meditation:** Practice gratitude meditation.

Sit in a quiet space, close your eyes, and think about the things you are grateful for and give thanks. Visualize each one in detail and feel the emotions associated with your gratitude. Gratitude meditation deepens your sense of appreciation.

8. **Gratitude for Challenges:** Shift your perspective on challenges. Instead of dwelling on the difficulty, reflect on the lessons and growth opportunities they offer. Express gratitude for the strength and resilience of these challenges that help you develop.

9. **Evening Reflection:** Before bedtime, reflect on the positive moments of your day. Acknowledge the small victories, moments of joy, and acts of kindness you experienced. Ending your day with gratitude can promote a sense of fulfillment.

By cultivating gratitude, you invite positivity and abundance into your life. Gratitude transforms your outlook, allowing you to focus on the blessings rather than the burdens. Embrace the practice of gratitude, and you will discover a deeper sense of contentment and joy.

Wishing you a day filled with gratitude and appreciation! □□

Day 29: Setting Intentions for Growth

Welcome to Day 29! As you approach the final days of this transformative experience, take some time today to set intentions for your ongoing growth and well- being. Intentions are powerful statements that reflect your aspirations and guide your actions. By setting clear intentions, you can align your focus and energy toward positive and meaningful goals.

Here is how to set intentions for your continued growth:

1. **Reflect on Your Journey:** Take a moment to reflect on the progress you've made during these 29 days.

Consider the positive changes, lessons learned, and challenges overcome. Acknowledge your strengths and resilience.

2. **Identify Areas for Growth:** Identify specific areas of your life where you would like to see growth and improvement. It could be related to your health, relationships, career, personal development, or any other aspect of your life. Be honest with yourself about what you truly desire.

3. **Formulate Positive Intentions:** Frame your intentions in positive, empowering language. Instead of focusing on what you want to avoid, state your intentions as positive affirmations. For example, "I am cultivating a healthy and balanced lifestyle" or "I am nurturing positive and supportive relationships."

Conclusion

4. **Be Specific and Realistic:** Make your intentions specific and realistic. Define clear actions or behaviors that align with your intentions. Setting achievable goals ensures that you can make steady progress toward your aspirations.

5. **Visualize Your Success:** Close your eyes and visualize yourself achieving your intentions. Imagine the feelings of accomplishment, fulfillment, and joy. Visualization can enhance your motivation and reinforce your commitment to your goals.

Conclusion

Day 30: Celebrating Your Achievements
Congratulations! You have reached Day 30 of your wellness journey, marking a significant milestone in your pursuit of well-being. Today is a day to celebrate your achievements, no matter how big or small. Take a moment to acknowledge your dedication, perseverance, and the positive changes you have made in the past 30 days. Here are some ways to celebrate your accomplishments:

1. **Reflect on Your Progress:** Take a moment to reflect on your journey. Consider the habits you have formed, the challenges you have overcome, and the lessons you've learned. Acknowledge your growth and the positive changes in your lifestyle.

2. **Practice Self-Appreciation:** Appreciate yourself for the efforts you have put into your well-being. Recognize your strengths, resilience, and commitment to your health and happiness. You can achieve remarkable things.

3. **Express Gratitude:** Express gratitude for the support you've received during your journey. Whether it is from friends, family, or online communities, acknowledging the people who have encouraged you can deepen your sense of connection and gratitude.

4. **Treat Yourself:** Treat yourself to something special as a reward for your achievements. It could be a relaxing spa day, a favorite meal, a movie night, or any activity that brings you joy. Celebrate your hard work with a well- deserved treat.

5. **Set New Goals:** Take this opportunity to set new goals for your continued well-being. Reflect on what you have learned and think about what you would like to accomplish next in your health journey. Set specific, realistic goals that align with your values and aspirations.

Conclusion

1. **Practice Mindfulness:** Be present in this moment and savor your achievements. Mindfully appreciate the progress you have made and the positive changes in your life. Mindfulness can deepen your sense of fulfillment.
2. **Share Your Success:** Share your achievements with others. Your journey may inspire and motivate others to embark on their wellness journeys. Celebrating together.
3. **Embrace Self-Love:** Embrace self-love and self-acceptance. You deserve love, respect, and kindness. Celebrate not only your external achievements but also your inner qualities and strengths. Remember, your wellness journey is ongoing, and each day presents new opportunities for growth and self-improvement.

By celebrating your achievements, you reinforce your positive habits and strengthen your commitment to your well-being. As you move forward, carry the sense of accomplishment from this 30-day journey with you, and continue to nurture your body, mind, and soul. Here is to your continued success and a future filled with health, happiness, and fulfillment! ☐☐☐

Conclusion
Conclusion: A Journey to Remember

As we reach the end of this transformative journey, it is essential to take a moment to reflect on how far we have come. Together, we've explored the depths of well-being, unraveling the threads that weave together the fabric of a fulfilling life. Along the way, we have embraced challenges, celebrated successes, and we have learned an irreplaceable lesson that true wellness is a holistic endeavor that encompasses body, mind, and soul.

In this exploration, we have discovered that wellness is not a destination but a way of living. It is a conscious choice to nourish our bodies with wholesome foods, to nurture our minds with positive thoughts, and to cultivate our spirits with gratitude and compassion. We have learned that self-care is not selfish; it is a prerequisite for giving our best to the world and to the people we love.

As you move forward from this journey, I encourage you to carry the lessons learned and the habits formed. Remember the power of mindfulness, the importance of self-compassion, and the transformative effects of gratitude. Continue to listen to your body, honor your emotions, and go after your passions and dreams. Always keep in mind that setbacks are not failures but opportunities for growth and resilience.

Conclusion

Conclusion: A Journey to Remember

The path to wellness is uniquely yours, and it may twist and turn, presenting unexpected challenges and delightful surprises. Embrace each twist and turn, for they are the markers of your personal growth and transformation. Surround yourself with positivity, seek support when needed, and never underestimate the impact of small, consistent steps toward your well-being. As you step out of these pages and back into the world, know that the journey doesn't end here—it continues with each mindful choice you make, each act of self-love, and each moment of gratitude. May your days be filled with vibrant health, profound joy, and a deep sense of fulfillment.

Thank you for allowing me to be a part of your wellness journey. Here is to a future brimming with vitality, purpose, and endless possibilities.

With Warmest Regards & Happy Juicing,
Chihauna

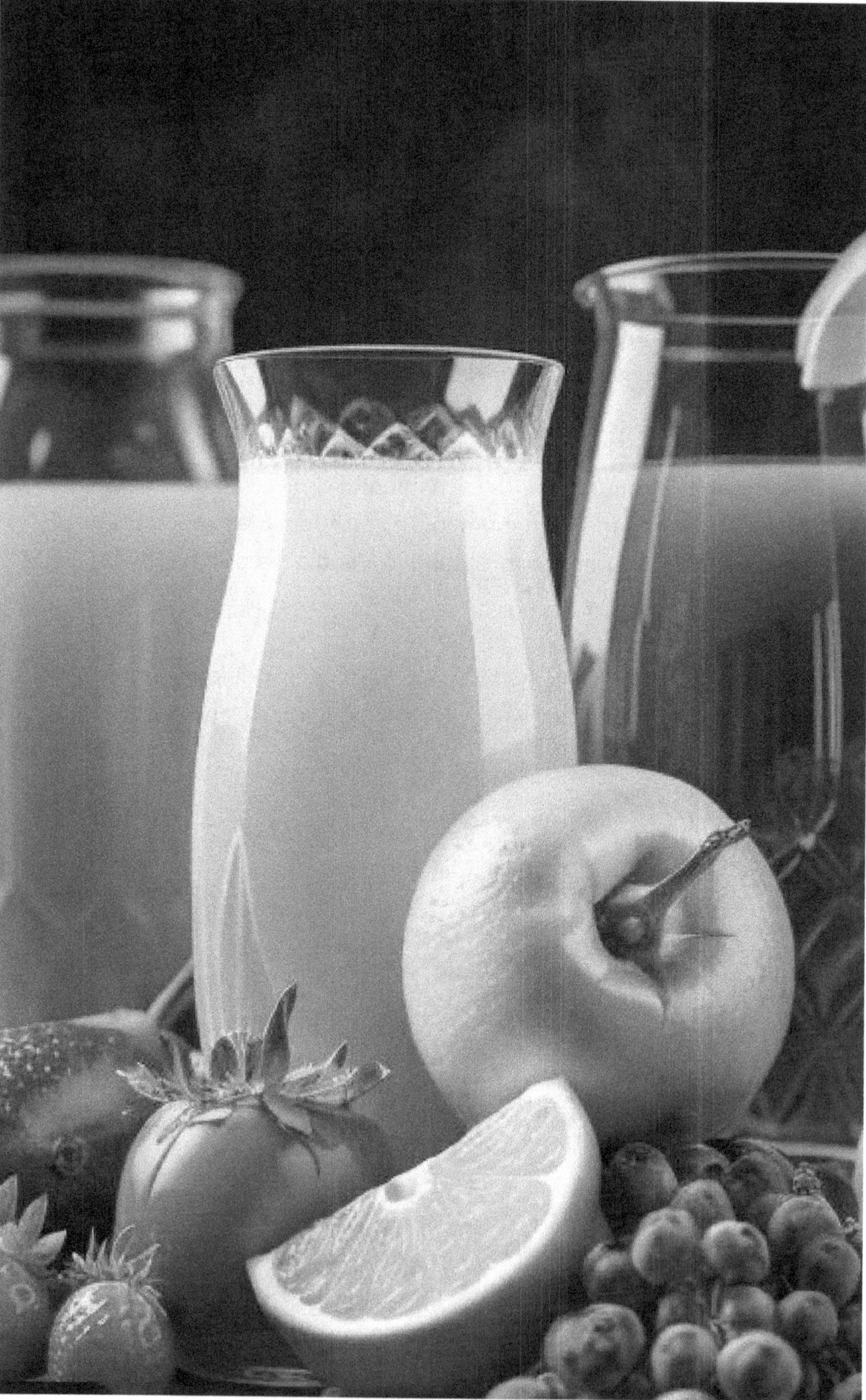